HODGKIN LYMPHOMA

A survival guide for patients

Dr. Bhratri Bhushan
MBBS, MD, DM

Copyright © 2021 Dr. Bhratri Bhushan

Copyright © 2021 by Dr. Bhratri Bhushan. All rights reserved. No part of this publication may be reproduced, distributed, or transmitted in any form or by any means, including photocopying, recording, or other electronic or mechanical methods, without the prior written permission of the publisher, except in the case of brief quotations embodied in critical reviews and certain other noncommercial uses permitted by copyright law. For permission requests, write to the publisher, addressed "Attention: Permissions Coordinator," at the address: A6, Jindal hospital, Hisar, Haryana, India 125001 www.bhratri@gmail.com This work is provided "as is," and the author and the publisher disclaim any and all warranties, express or implied, including any warranties as to accuracy, comprehensiveness, or currency of the content of this work. This work is no substitute for individual patient assessment based on healthcare professionals' examination of each patient and consideration of, among other things, age, weight, gender, current or prior medical conditions, medication history, laboratory data, and other factors unique to the patient. The publisher does not provide medical advice or guidance, and this work is merely a reference tool. Healthcare professionals, and not the publisher, are solely responsible for the use of this work including all medical judgments and for any resulting diagnosis and treatments. Given continuous, rapid advances in medical science and health information, independent professional verification of medical diagnoses, indications, appropriate pharmaceutical selections and dosages, and treatment options should be made and healthcare professionals should consult a variety of sources. When prescribing medication, healthcare professionals are advised to consult the product information sheet (the manufacturer's package insert) accompanying each drug to verify, among other things, conditions of use, warnings, and side effects and identify any changes in dosage schedule or contraindications, particularly if the medication to be administered is new, infrequently used, or has a narrow therapeutic range. To the maximum extent permitted under applicable law, no responsibility is assumed by the publisher for any injury and/or damage to persons or property as a matter of products liability, negligence law or otherwise, or from any reference to or use by any person of this work.

CONTENTS

Title Page
Copyright
Preface
Hodgkin lymphoma 1
About The Author 45

PREFACE

Hodgkin lymphoma is one of the most treatable cancers. With the advent of new diagnostic and therapeutic modalities, the management landscape of Hodgkin lymphoma has dramatically changed. In this book, together we will explore the subject of Hodgkin lymphoma. This will help you understand the disease better. It is overwhelming to know that either you or your loved one has been diagnosed with Hodgkin lymphoma and it may sound unrealistic that at this trying time you should pick up a book and understand the disease biology and management strategies but believe me, it is important. Today all of the decision making in medicine, especially in oncology, is "shared" decision making. What it means is that the team treating you is just one part of the decision making process, the other part is you and your family. An informed decision is a good decision and to make an informed decision, you must have reasonably enough knowledge of the subject.

The goal of this book is in no way to be an all

encompassing, comprehensive reference for all of your questions; but to provide you all of the useful information, without unnecessarily burdening you with confusing facts and figures. I have constructed this book in an interactive format, i.e., questions and answers. Most of these question I have picked up by my daily encounters with patients and their families and some I have constructed myself to bridge the gaps between the topics. I hope you will find this book helpful. I wish you and your loved ones long, healthy and prosperous lives.

HODGKIN LYMPHOMA

Q. What is Hodgkin lymphoma?

Answer: our bodies have the lymphatic system, which is basically a network of lymph nodes and interconnecting lymph vessels. The lymphatic system is made up of many organs: lymph nodes, lymph vessels, spleen, thymus and bone marrow. One of the major functions of the lymphatic system is to fight infections.

There are many kinds of cells, which are stored in the organs that are parts of the lymphatic system. Lymphocytes (a type of white blood cells) are cells that are a major part of our lymphatic system. Lymphocytes are mainly of two types: B cells and T cells.

Cancer of lymphocytes in known as lymphoma. Hodgkin lymphoma (HL), formerly called Hodgkin's disease, is a type of lymphoma. HL originates from the B cells, specifically "mature" B cells. There are many other types of lymphomas as well, for example diffuse large B cell lymphoma, follicular lymphoma, mantle cell lymphoma etc. The name "Hodgkin lymphoma" was given in the honour of Thomas Hodgkin, who published the first case report of this cancer in 1832.

Note that Hodgkin lymphoma (HL) is not just of one type. There are many types of HL that are identified by certain tests. You may encounter terms like classical HL, nodular sclerosis HL, mixed cellularity HL, nodular lymphocyte predominant HL etc. This classification of HL not only helps in formulation of the best treatment plan but also in prognostication.

HL develops when the lymphocytes become abnormal (cancerous) and their normal patterns of proliferation are disrupted. This leads to uncontrollable growth of the abnormal lymphocytes which then travel to different parts of the body and may accumulate in lymph nodes. This leads to myriads of symptoms and signs, one of which is swelling of lymph nodes, medically known as lymphadenopathy.

Please note that not all lymphomas are HL. HL is just one type of lymphoma. HL is basically of two types: classical HL (CHL) and nodular lymphocyte-predominant HL (NLPHL).

Q. Why have I developed HL?

Answer: there are some cancers for which a causative agent or factor, also called etiologic agent, is known. For example, cigarette smoking is a risk factor for lung cancer, HPV infection is a risk factor for cervical cancer etc. Note that an etiologic agent is not only associated with a cancer but also has epidemiologic significance. What I mean is that there may be very rare causes of certain cancers, which may well explain the occurrence of a cancer in some people but their association with cancer can not be generalised.

The etiology of HL is not entirely clear, for most of the cases there is no known cause. There are many factors linked with the development of HL but there is not a single, "definite" etiologic agent associated with it. Epstein-Barr virus (EBV) infection plays a role in some cases of HL.

Note the following points:
1. HL is not an inherited disease. In other words, relatives and children of patients with HL **are not at an increased risk** of developing HL. Some patients with HL may have a family history of HL or some other lymphoma in one or more of their family members, but based on the presently available data, it is entirely coincidental.
2. HL more commonly affects young people. HL has two incidence peaks (a "bimodal"

age distribution): one is young adults and one in persons older than 50 years.
3. In the adolescent age group, females are more commonly affected by HL; on the other hand, in children under 5 years of age, HL affects boys more commonly than girls.

Q. What are the symptoms of HL?

Answer: HL can present in many ways, the most common presenting symptom is a painless, enlarged lymph node. The enlarged lymph node is most commonly present in the neck, but may also be found in the armpit, groin or above the collar bone. The lymph nodes affected by HL usually have a "rubbery" consistency (they are not very hard). Lymph nodes are present in almost all parts of our bodies and any of the lymph nodes may become enlarged due to HL. If nodes inside the chest (mediastinal lymph nodes) become enlarged, then they may cause tightness in chest, cough, difficulty breathing etc. If lymph nodes in the abdomen become enlarged, then depending on their location, may give rise to myriads of symptoms, for example, abdominal fullness, enlarged spleen (spleen in a lymphatic organ), early satiety, pain etc.

There are some symptoms that are of particular importance, both diagnostically and prognostically. These symptoms are known as "B symptoms". If these symptoms are present, please consult your doctor and even if you consult a doctor for an enlarged lymph node (lump) in your neck, groin etc., you should tell your doctor if any of these symptoms is present. The "B symptoms" are:

1. Fever
2. Night sweats
3. Weight loss: unexplained weight loss exceeding 10% of body weight during the 6 months prior to diagnosis.

In advanced stage, HL may infiltrate bone marrow and cause anemia, increased rates of infection and bleeding.

In some countries, tuberculosis is endemic. The signs/symptoms of HL may mimic those of TB.

Remember that if you have an enlarged lymph node in your neck (or any other area), most of the time it's due to an infective cause rather than cancer, but it is imperative to consult a doctor for proper evaluation.

Q. How is HL diagnosed?

Answer: the most important step in the diagnosis of HL is biopsy of an affected lymph node or organ. It is preferable to remove the whole of the suspected lymph node (excisional biopsy), however if excisional biopsy is not possible, then a part of lymph node may be removed (incisional biopsy). Whenever possible, biopsy is done under local anesthesia; but if the lymph node or the affected organ is deeper, general anesthesia may be required.

The biopsy specimen (tissue) is studied under a microscope and specialised tests, for example immunohistochemistry, are performed to reach a proper diagnosis.

Note that the question was "how is HL diagnosed?", and the answer is "by microscopic examination of the tissue obtained by biopsy". There is no other way to diagnose HL, biopsy is mandatory.

Q. Are there stages of HL?

Answer: Yes, there are stages. I would like to stress here that the stages of HL are not the same as the stages of, say, lung cancer. For example, if lung cancer is diagnosed in the fourth stage, there are virtually no chances of complete cure and the intent of treatment is palliative. On the other hand, if HL is diagnosed in the fourth stage, it means that the disease will be harder to control than the earlier stages and chances of relapse are higher after attaining remission, but the designation of stage four in HL **does not** mean that the disease is incurable. This should be kept in mind. I routinely encounter this problem in my practice: When I tell my patients that they are suffering from stage IV HL, they tend to lose hope, thinking that the cancer has spread beyond control. That is not the case. Period.

The staging workup may be somewhat different for different patients, depending on the clinical situation. Basically, following are the steps involved in proper staging of HL:

1. History and physical exam: this is the simplest step, in which a doctor inquires a patient about the symptoms, their duration etc. A physical examination is then conducted, which primarily focuses on the lymph node regions. A doctor will palpate (touch) various areas of the body and look for abnormal findings. Routine physical examination, like listening to heart sounds and respiratory sounds et cetera is also a part of comprehensive physical examination. A physical examination not only helps in determining the extent of the disease but also in guiding further, specialised tests.
2. Blood tests are performed in all patients. A complete blood count, comprehensive metabolic panel, viral markers and other tests are part of the blood tests.
3. Bone marrow biopsy is done to look for bone marrow infiltration. In some cases, bone marrow biopsy may not be necessary, but that depends on the judgment of the

clinician.
4. PET-CT scan: it is perhaps the most informative staging test for HL. Please note that whenever possible, a PET-CT scan is a must. If PET-CT is not possible, CT scan may be utilised, but it doesn't provide the critical "metabolic" information that PET-CT provides.

Now let's go though some basics of staging:
1. The staging workup (using the tests described above) is an exercise for determining the extent of the disease.
2. The staging of HL depends on the number of lymph node regions involved, whether or not lymph node regions are affected on the both sides of the diaphragm and involvement of other organs, lymphatic or nonlymphatic.

The four stage groups of HL are as follows:
1. Stage I: Only one lymph node region is involved, only one lymph structure is involved, or only one extranodal site (IE) is involved.
2. Stage II: Two or more lymph node regions or lymph node structures on the **same side** of the diaphragm are involved.
3. Stage III: Lymph node regions or structures on **both sides** of the diaphragm are involved.

4. Stage IV: There is widespread involvement of a number of organs or tissues other than lymph node regions or structures, such as the liver, lung, or bone marrow.

Further, after the stage, a letter, either A or B, is mentioned; for example stage IIA or IIIB.
1. "A" means that fever, weight loss, and night sweats are **not** present.
2. "B" means that fever, weight loss, or night sweats are present.

Q. How is HL treated?

Answer: Hodgkin lymphoma is one of the most prominent success stories of modern day cancer therapy. It is one of the most treatable forms of cancer. With the initial treatment, More than 75 percent of patients can be cured and 10 year survival rates exceed 90%. For the purpose of treatment planning, HL is divided into two groups:
1. Classical HL (CHL)
2. Nodular lymphocyte-predominant HL (NLPHL)

This classification is based on the microscopic and immunohistochemistry examination of tumor tissue obtained by biopsy.

In this section we will discuss the management of

CHL. The management of NLPHL will be discussed at the end of this book.

CHL is of four types: nodular sclerosis, mixed cellularity, lymphocyte rich and lymphocyte depleted. The management of these four types of CHL is similar. As we have discussed in the previous question, there are four stages of HL. For the purpose of treatment planning, CHL is divided into two groups:
1. Early stage (stage I and stage II)
2. Advanced stage (stage III and stage IV)

Generally, early stage CHL is treated with chemotherapy followed by radiation therapy or chemotherapy alone; whereas advanced stage CHL is treated with chemotherapy alone or sometimes, chemotherapy followed by radiation therapy.

Q. How is early stage HL treated?

Answer: combination of chemotherapy and radiation therapy is used for treatment of early stage (stage I and II) CHL. The prognosis of early stage HL is excellent, complete cure is possible in almost all patient with the initial treatment. The combined use of chemotherapy and radiation therapy in early stage CHL results in higher response rates and higher chances of long term cure compared with chemotherapy alone. However, the combined use of chemo and radiation may result in higher chances of long term side effects. Sometimes, only chemo may be used (without any radiation therapy). In summary, generally, early stage CHL is treated by chemotherapy followed by radiation therapy.

Chemotherapy:
1. A combination of several chemotherapy drugs is used for the treatment of early stage CHL. Such combinations of chemotherapy drugs are called "regimens". The most commonly used chemotherapy regimen for early stage CHL is a combination of four drugs (ABVD):
    1. Doxorubicin (A)
    2. Bleomycin (B)
    3. Vinblastine (V)
    4. Dacarbazine (D)
2. All of these four drugs are given into a vein (intravenously). The chemotherapy regimen also has some oral medicines that are given to reduce side effects of chemo.
3. All of these four drugs are given on the same day and the next session is given 14 days later. Two such sessions make up one "cycle" of treatment. So, if you are planned for three cycles of ABVD, you will have to take chemo six times, each session being 14 days apart.

We will discuss the side effects of chemotherapy later.

Radiation therapy:
1. A machine (most commonly, a linear accelerator) is used for deliver high-energy X-rays, also known as radiation therapy. Radiation therapy is recommended in many stage I and II CHL patients.
2. Generally, for the treatment of CHL, chemo is given first and then radiation is given. Alternatively, chemotherapy alone may be used and in such cases, radiation is not used at all.
3. Radiation therapy is given daily (five days per week) for many weeks.
4. Nowadays, the techniques of radiation therapy have evolved. ISRT (involved site radiation therapy) or INRT (involved nodal radiation therapy) have replaced large field RT, which has resulted in decreased side effects.

We will discuss about the side effects of radiation therapy later.

Go through the following points very carefully:
1. The prognosis of early stage CHL is excellent. Almost all of the patients achieve complete cure with the initial treatment and long term survival is the norm.
2. Chemotherapy followed by radiation therapy offers the highest chances of long term cure in early stage CHL. However, the combined use of chemo and radiation is associated with higher chances of long term side

effects than chemotherapy alone.
3. Sometimes, only chemotherapy is used for the treatment of early stage CHL.
4. Note that while **chemo alone is an option** for the treatment of early early stage CHL, **radiation alone is not an option**. Radiation is always given in combination with (following) chemotherapy for the treatment of early stage CHL.
5. The choice between chemo followed by radiation and chemo alone depends on many factors. Please discuss about the pros and cons of both of these options in your case with your oncologist.
6. ABVD is the most commonly used regimen for the treatment of early stage CHL.

Q. How is advanced stage CHL treated?

Answer: advanced stage (stage III and IV) CHL is treated with chemotherapy. As we have discussed in the previous question, for early stage HL, radiation therapy is often combined with chemotherapy, but **for advanced stage CHL, radiation therapy is not routinely used**; its use is restricted to specific situations in advanced stage CHL.

The most commonly used regimen for advanced stage CHL is ABVD. There are other regimens available for the treatment of advanced HL. The choice among the recommended regimens depends on clinical factors, preference of the clinician and institutional practices. Ask your doctor about the various regimens and their pros and cons.

Chemotherapy:
1. A combination of several chemotherapy drugs is used for the treatment of advanced stage CHL. Such combinations of chemotherapy are called "regimens". The most commonly used chemotherapy regimen for advanced stage CHL is a combination of four drugs (ABVD):
    1. Doxorubicin (A)
    2. Bleomycin (B)
    3. Vinblastine (V)
    4. Dacarbazine (D)
2. All of these four drugs are given into a vein (intravenously). The chemotherapy regimen also has some oral medicines that are given to reduce side effects of chemo.
3. All of these four drugs are given on the same day and the next session is given 14 days later. Two such sessions make up one "cycle" of treatment. So, if you are planned for six cycles of ABVD, you will have to take chemo twelve times, each session being 14 days apart.
4. There are other options available for the treatment of advanced stage CHL. The options include:

1. A+AVD: this regimen has four drugs in it, Doxorubicin, Brentuximab vedotin, Vinblastine and Dacarbazine. This regimen in similar to ABVD, but instead of bleomycin, it uses brentuximab vedotin. Bleomycin is not a good drug for patients with lung problems, thus, in patients with lung problems A+AVD can be used instead of ABVD.
2. Stanford V: it includes doxorubicin, vinblastine, mechlorethamine, etoposide, vincristine, bleomycin and prednisone. Note that Stanford V regimen includes radiation therapy.
3. BEACOPP: it includes bleomycin, etoposide, doxorubicin, cyclophosphamide, vincristine, procarbazine and prednisone. This regimen is associated with higher incidence of toxicity compared with ABVD. BEACOPP is more commonly used in Europe.

More facts about chemotherapy in advanced HL:
1. Escalated BEACOPP has greater efficacy than ABVD in patients up to 60 years old.
2. Escalated BEACOPP–treated patients experience more toxicity compared with ABVD-treated patients.
3. Using six rather than eight cycles of escal-

ated BEACOPP may reduce toxicity without compromising outcomes.
4. Almost 70% of patients with advanced HL will be cured with ABVD, so it is not necessary to choose a toxic regimen such as escalated BEACOPP for all patients with advanced HL. The choice between ABVD and other, more intensive regimens depends on many factors. Please have a thorough discussion with your oncologist in this regard.

You may hear terms like "escalation" of therapy. This is a relatively new practice. Let's understand this by an example: Suppose that a patient has been diagnosed with stage III or IV HL (stage III and IV are advanced stage HL), and he's started on ABVD regimen. After 2 cycles (4 chemo administrations, each 14 days apart), a PET-CT is done. If PET-CT reveals a good response, then ABVD is continued; however if the PET-CT results are not suggestive of a good response, then a more intense regimen than ABVD may be used. This form of adjustment is known as escalation of therapy. The logic behind this approach is that if PET-CT doesn't show a good response after 2 cycles of ABVD, then chances are that the disease might not get cured with ABVD alone, even after 6 cycles.

Another approach is de-escalation, in which a more intense regimen than ABVD is initially stated and if PET-CT shows good response after 2 cycles, then the intensity of that regimen may be reduced or ABVD might be started.

The decision of changing the regimen depends on many factors, and experts have different opinions in this regard. However, PET-CT should be done after every 2 cycles of any chemotherapy for HL, in my opinion.

Radiation therapy:
1. Radiation therapy is not routinely used for the treatment of advanced CHL.
2. Radiation therapy, whenever used, is given after completion of planned course of chemotherapy.
3. In the following scenarios, radiation therapy may be considered in advanced CHL:
    1. If the cancer was "bulky" at presentation.
    2. If the cancer doesn't completely disappear with chemotherapy.

Q. What are the side effects of chemotherapy in patients with HL?

Answer: chemotherapy protocols used for treatment of HL have different drugs, dosages and combination thereof. The toxicity profile of a regimen depends on the drugs being used, their doses, frequency of administration and patient-related factors, like overall health, comorbidities, organ functions, phase of the treatment etc.

Some side effects of chemo are seen in almost all patients and most of the side effects are temporary and resolve either on their own or with medical treatment. There are some long-term effects of chemo as well, the incidence, severity and timing of which can not be predicted with certainty. The risk of long-term and irreversible side effects is always there but statistically, the benefits of chemo in HL far outweigh its potential side effects.

The common side effects are:
1. Nausea
2. Vomiting
3. Constipation or diarrhea
4. Hair loss
5. Fatigue
6. Loss of appetite
7. Increased risk of infections
8. Numbness/tingling or other nervous system side effects.

Serious side effects, which are seen only in some of the patients, include:
1. Heart problems: doxorubicin is primarily responsible for heart problems. There is a "ceiling" dose of doxorubicin that should not be exceeded. In the treatment of HL, doxorubicin is used in such a manner that

this ceiling dose is respected. Thus, in most patients there are no long-term heart problems. If you have a heart condition, then your chances of having such side effects may be higher.
2. Lung problems: bleomycin is primarily responsible for lung problems, which may sometimes be very serious. A test, known as DLCO (along with other lung function tests), is done periodically (ideally before each cycle) to detect the lung damage early and if lung damage is found, then bleomycin may be discontinued depending on the clinical situation. If you already have a lung disease, then choosing a regimen without bleomycin may be a better option.
3. Infertility: ABVD is generally considered a safe regimen as far as fertility is concerned. On the other hand, BEACOPP is associated with ovarian failure in women and decreased sperm count in men. If you are of childbearing age, then please discuss about the fertility preservation options with your healthcare provider.
4. Long term survivors of HL are more likely to develop second cancers. Breast cancer, lung cancer and blood cancer are some of the cancers, incidence of which may be increased in HL survivors. You may have to undergo screening for some of these cancers after your treatment has been com-

pleted. Please ask your doctor more about second cancers, their prevention and measures for their timely detection.

Q. What are the side effects of radiation therapy in patients with HL?

Answer: in the past, radiation therapy for HL was given to very large areas of body and it was associated with many short-term and long-term side effects. With the advancement of radiation therapy technology, nowadays the radiation exposure to unaffected areas can be limited and thus, the incidence of side effects has been reduced significantly.

Side effects of radiation therapy in HL include:
1. Skin damage: skin color may change and a burning sensation may be felt.
2. Sore throat
3. Difficulty in swallowing
4. Alteration or loss of taste
5. Nausea, vomiting

Long term side effects on radiation therapy may include development of second cancers, heart problems, lung problems etc. The incidence of breast cancer may be increased later in life in young females receiving radiation therapy to chest. These long-term side effects are seen only in a minority of patients. Please discuss about the anticipated side effects of radiation, their prevention and management with your radiation oncologist.

Q. What are my chances of cure?

Answer: the key word here is "chances"; in other words, prognosis is not a certainty, only a probability. I often tell my patients that statistics are more useful for oncologists than patients, because a patient will either be completely cured or not. I know that it's not an adequate explanation, what I want to convey is that don't get disheartened by looking at the 5-year survival rates and 3-year relapse free survival rates etc. Some patients get too caught up in numbers, thereby adding to their levels of distress. Fortunately, HL is one of the most curable cancer. Note the following points about chances of cure in HL:
1. In early-stage HL, the use of combined-modality treatment (chemotherapy followed by radiation therapy) produces the best results. Almost all patients are cured and 10 year survival rates are more than 90%.
2. Note that around 90% of patients of early-stage HL can be cured with chemotherapy alone, and since radiation therapy may be associated with long-term side effects, especially when given in adolescence or young age, a chemotherapy alone approach may be chosen for some patients with early-

stage HL.

3. Advanced stage HL is treated with chemotherapy, and in some circumstances radiation therapy may be given as consolidation therapy. However, complete remissions after initial therapy are not achieved in approximately 20% of patients with stage III or IV HL (in other words, complete remissions are achieved in around 80% of patients with stage III or IV HL) with the initial treatment. Patients who don't achieve complete response fare poorly than those who do.

4. Long-term survival in advanced stage HL is not as good. There are models available for prediction of long term survival in advanced HL. The most commonly used model is the IPS, or International Prognostic Score, model. The discussion of IPS is out of the scope of this book. Please discuss more about it with your oncologist.

Q. I have completed therapy for HL. How will the response of therapy be evaluated? How can I be sure that the HL is gone?

Answer: After completion of the course of treatment, response evaluation is done.

Following are the components of the response evaluation:

1. Medical history
2. Physical examination
3. Blood tests
4. And most importantly, a PET-CT.

Note that the PET-CT is usually done:
1. Six to eight weeks after finishing chemotherapy (if only chemotherapy was used for treatment) OR
2. Eight to twelve weeks after finishing radiation therapy.

The goal of HL treatment is "CR" or complete response, also called complete remission. The definition of CR requires that all of the following criteria are met:
1. History and physical examination reveal no evidence of disease or disease-related symptoms.
2. There is no "increased uptake" on PET. This requires some explanation. If we only do a CT scan (without PET), it may still show some lymph nodes which are enlarged (abnormal), after the completion of treatment. But these abnormal appearing lymph nodes may not have residual cancer in them. Doing a PET-CT not only provides us the anatomic details of lymph nodes, and other organs, but also the "uptake" within them. If the lymph nodes (or any other abnormal growth) "light up" on a PET-CT, it means

that cancer is still present and if they don't light up, it means that the abnormality is only anatomical, there is no residual cancer.
3. If a bone marrow biopsy was done before starting treatment and it was positive, then it should be negative to be classified as complete response.

Q. I have achieved complete response after my planned course of treatment. What should be done next?

Answer: congratulations, you have achieved CR, now your treatment is complete. Note that:
1. There is no role of any maintenance therapy after CR in HL. You don't need to take any drugs, for HL, once the planned course has been completed and you have achieved CR.
2. For HL, there is no role of stem cell transplant, also colloquially called BMT, in the first CR.

What you do have to go through is surveillance. Surveillance is done for two basic reasons:
1. To monitor treatment complications.
2. To detect possible relapse.

The frequency of visits is not strictly defined, it depends on the clinical situation and the preference of the doctor and the patient. History and physical examination are a must at every visit but the role of imaging tests is not very significant.

Remember:
1. Performing CT scans very frequently is not likely to impact outcomes in case of relapse. Besides, CT scans lead to radiation exposure, which leads to more harm than good in long term. Studies show that relapse is often first detected based on symptoms and physical examination findings rather than CT scans.
2. PET-CT or PET alone has no role in long term surveillance of otherwise healthy patients on follow up.

A point to remember here is that most cases of relapse occur within the first two years of completion of treatment. So, that's the time the patients have to be very vigilant of any symptoms. After two years, the chances of relapse fall, although surveillance is still continued with increasing intervals.

Q. I have completed my planned course of treatment, but the doctors told me that I haven't achieved a complete response. What does it mean and what should I do next?

Answer: the goal is to achieve complete response, but if CR is not achieved, it is not good news. If CR is not achieved then the HL is considered "refractory". Please remember that no matter how little is the disease burden still present after completion of treatment, it has to be considered refractory and must be treated with second line therapy; in other words, there is no "wait-and-watch" approach for its management. We will discuss the treatment of refractory HL later.

Q. What is the role of bone marrow transplantation (stem cell transplantation) in the treatment of HL?

Answer: remember these three facts about stem cell transplantation in HL:
1. There is **no role** of stem cell transplantation patients with HL who achieve complete remission with initial treatment.
2. If the initial treatment fails to produce a complete remission, then stem cell transplantation may be done.
3. If the HL comes back after complete remission, stem cell transplantation may be done.

If you are a candidate (according to your oncologist) for stem cell transplantation, please go through this book of mine, it may be of some help to you: https://www.amazon.com/dp/B099TSBMYW

Q. What if my HL comes back?

Answer: as we have already discussed, long-term survival rates are excellent in HL, but in some patients relapse occurs. Relapsed HL is harder to treat. There are some patients, who don't achieve complete response with the initial treatment, their HL is considered "refractory". If you are suffering from a refractory or relapsed HL, then please understand that cure is still possible. There are following options for the treatment of relapsed/refractory HL:
1. Additional chemotherapy with a new regimen.
2. Stem cell transplantation.
3. Targeted therapy.
4. Immunotherapy.

The treatment decision making in relapsed/refractory HL is a highly complex subject and there is no one-size-fits-all approach. In my opinion, if you are fit enough to undergo a stem cell transplantation procedure, then it's the best option.
Note that stem cell transplantation is relapsed HL is generally performed by using your own stem cells, you will not need a donor (an autologous transplant). However, in some cases stem cells procured from a donor are used (an allogeneic transplant).

Some facts about treatment of relapsed/refractory HL:
1. Chemotherapy (there are many regimens)

is started first. If the patient responds to chemo and he/she is fit enough, high-dose chemotherapy and bone marrow transplant is the best option. The bone marrow transplant here refers to "autologous hematopoietic stem cell transplantation". Please note that this type of transplant uses the stem cells of the patient him/herself (a donor is not required).

2. If stem cell transplantation is not possible, then targeted therapy or immunotherapy are options.
3. If stem cell transplantation, targeted therapy or immunotherapy are not possible, then palliative chemotherapy is an option. There are many regimens available for the treatment of relapsed/refractory HL.
4. Sometimes, no active treatment is chosen and only palliative care is continued.

In my opinion, if a clinical trial is available, then relapsed/refractory HL patients must get enrolled in it. Ask your doctor for more information.

Q. What is nodular lymphocyte-predominant HL (NLPHL)? How is it treated?

Answer: there are two types on HL: classical HL (which is of four types, discussed in the previous questions) and NLPHL. Nodular lymphocyte-predominant Hodgkin lymphoma (NLPHL) is an uncommon subtype of HL. It is generally a slower growing lymphoma than CHL.

The diagnostic work-up and staging of both of these types of HL are similar, but treatment protocols are different.

For treatment planning, NLPHL is divided into the following categories:
1. Non-bulky **early stage** NLPHL (stage I or II, non-bulky): these patients don't have any of the characteristics of bulky or non-contiguous **early stage** NLPHL.
2. Bulky or non-contiguous **early stage** NLPHL: patients having ≥10 cm tumor mass or non-contiguous disease or disease-related symptoms or organ-threatening mass.
3. Advanced NLPHL: Stage III or stage IV NLPHL.

Important points about treatment of NLPHL:
1. Non-bulky early stage NLPHL:
    1. Not all patients with non-bulky early stage NLPHL require treatment, some patient may just undergo active surveillance without any treatment.
    2. Some patients are treated with involved-site radiation therapy (ISRT).
    3. Chemotherapy is **not** generally used

for the treatment of non-bulky early stage NLPHL.
2. Bulky or non-contiguous early stage NLPHL:
    1. These patients require treatment. For them, active surveillance is not a good option.
    2. They can be treated with either chemoimmunotherapy alone or ISRT alone. Combination of chemoimmunotherapy followed by ISRT is **not used** for treatment of bulky or non-contiguous early stage NLPHL.
    3. R-CHOP regimen (a combination of rituximab, cyclophosphamide, doxorubicin, vincristine and prednisone) is the most commonly used chemoimmunotherapy regimen.
    4. Some patients are not candidates for ISRT or chemoimmunotherapy (R-CHOP regimen) (due to frailty, comorbidities or contraindications); for these patients, following are the options;
        1. Single-agent rituximab
        2. Active surveillance
3. Advanced NLPHL (stage III or IV NLPHL):
    1. Not all patients with advanced NLPHL require treatment. Some of the patients with advanced NLPHL may be started on active surveillance

alone, without any treatment.
2. For the purpose of treatment planning, patients with advanced NLPHL are divided into two groups:
    1. Asymptomatic or minimally symptomatic
    2. Symptomatic
3. Asymptomatic or minimally symptomatic:
    1. Some patients with advanced NLPHL have either no symptoms or have only minimal symptoms. Also, to be classified under this category, a patient must not have any "organ threatening masses".
    2. There are three options for the treatment of such patients:
        1. Chemoimmunotherapy (R-CHOP)
        2. Single-agent rituximab
        3. Active surveillance (it is the preferred approach for most of the patients).
4. Symptomatic:
    1. Some patients with advanced NLPHL have symptoms or organ threatening masses.
    2. There are the following options for such patients (the choice among these options

depends on many factors):
1. Chemoimmunotherapy (R-CHOP)
2. ISRT
3. Chemoimmunotherapy followed by ISRT

Remember:
1. Not all patients with NLPHL require treatment.
2. Patients with NLPHL who do require treatment can be managed by a variety of strategies depending on the clinical situation:

   1. Chemoimmunotherapy

   2. ISRT

   3. Chemoimmunotherapy followed by ISRT
3. RCHOP is the most commonly used protocol for treatment of NLPHL, there are other options also, eg, R-CVP, R-ABVD. For the treatment of NLPHL, usually 6 cycles of R-CHOP are given. If combined modality therapy is being used, lesser cycles of R-CHOP may be used.
4. Radiation therapy may be used in combination with R-CHOP chemoimmunotherapy for treatment of NLPHL.
5. Some notes on radiation therapy for localised NLPHL:

   1. Radiation therapy uses high-energy X-rays to kill cancer cells. It is

delivered by a machine.

2. Radiation therapy is started once the cycles of RCHOP chemoimmunotherapy have been completed. Some patients may be treated with only radiation therapy (without any chemotherapy).

3. Radiation therapy is given daily, for five days per week successively (followed by 2 days rest). Generally, three to five weeks of radiation therapy is given for the treatment of localised NLPHL. Your radiation oncologist may choose a different schedule, depending on the clinical situation.

4. Generally, in NLPHL, radiation therapy is well tolerated and side effects are minimal and manageable. Please ask your doctors about the pros and cons, and expected side effects of radiation therapy in your case.

Some notes on chemoimmunotherapy:
1. Chemotherapy are drugs, which kill cancer cells but are not specific; in other words, they also kill normal cells to some degree. The cells which are rapidly dividing are killed preferentially by chemotherapy drugs.

2. Immunotherapy means targeted therapy in form of monoclonal antibodies. The cancerous cells of NLPHL have molecules on their surface, most notably CD20, which can be targeted by immunotherapy drugs. I would like to clarify here that immunotherapy may be of many types, and for the purpose of initial treatment of NLPHL, the anti-CD20 monoclonal antibody rituximab is used.

The most commonly used chemoimmunotherapy, for the treatment of NLPHL is: R-CHOP. This regimen has five drugs in it:
1. Rituximab (R)
2. Cyclophosphamide (C)
3. Doxorubicin (H)
4. Vincristine (O)
5. Prednisone (P)

In case you are wondering, doxorubicin is written as "H" because the chemical name of doxorubicin is hydroxydaunorubicin and vincristine is also called oncovin, so it is written as "O".

Note here that:
1. R is immunotherapy (monoclonal antibody).
2. CHOP is chemotherapy.

Important points about R-CHOP protocol:

1. R, C, H and O are given into a vein (intravenously).
2. R, C, H and O are given successively over the course of one day.
3. The fifth drug, P (prednisone) is given by mouth (in tablet form). Prednisone is given for five days.
4. The next cycle is given three weeks later. In other words, cycles are repeated every 3 weeks.
5. This regimen is generally given for 6 cycles, sometimes 8 cycles may given.
6. Note that the administration of chemotherapy is not the most difficult part, it's very straightforward and apart from mild infusion related effects, not much is to be expected on the very first day. Side effects arise over the course of ensuing weeks.
7. Side effects:
    1. Side effects are commonly observed with RCHOP regimen.
    2. As we have already discussed, chemotherapy primarily affects rapidly dividing cells. Cancer cells of NLPHL are rapidly dividing, so they are obviously affected. But there are many other cells in our body that are rapidly dividing, for example blood cells, cells of gastrointestinal tract lining, cells in the hair follicles etc. These cells are also killed by chemo-

therapy, accounting for many side effects.

3. Chemo results in lowering of neutrophils (a type of white blood cells), it is to be expected. The medical term of decreased neutrophil counts is "neutropenia". Some amount of neutropenia is found in almost all of the patients treated with RCHOP at some point in time during the course. Sometimes, fever may be associated with neutropenia, a condition known as febrile neutropenia. Please remember that febrile neutropenia (FN) is a medical emergency, so if a patient experiences fever (in this case, defined as temperature of 100.4°F or more), medical help must immediately be sought. Usually, all patients with febrile neutropenia require admission and antibiotic administration.

4. Other blood cells may also be decreased. If RBCs decrease below a certain level, it manifests as anemia. If platelets fall below a certain threshold, thrombocytopenia may result. Not all patients with anemia or thrombocytopenia require treatment, it depends on a variety of factors.

5. Another common side effect is nausea and/or vomiting. Nausea and/or vomiting may develop in 30 to 90% of patients treated with RCHOP. Medicines for prevention or reduction of severity of nausea and vomiting are standard parts of the RCHOP regimen. Drugs like dexamethasone, 5-HT3 antagonists (like ondansetron) and aprepitant are commonly used for this purpose.
6. Although almost all drugs used in the RCHOP regimen may give rise to hypersensitivity reactions, rituximab is most commonly associated with these reactions. These reactions most commonly occur in the very first cycle, however, they may occur in the later cycles as well. Hypersensitivity reactions manifest as flushing itching, chest, back, or abdominal pain fever, nausea dizziness etc. Not all patients experience these reactions. Generally these reactions are mild and easily subside but they may be severe. Drugs are given routinely before chemoimmunotherapy to prevent or reduce these reactions. Drugs like acetaminophen, diphenhydramine, hydrocortisone and famotidine are used for this purpose.

7. Tumor lysis syndrome: it is a potentially life-threatening condition which results from rapid death of tumor cells and release of toxic substances from these dying cells. Preventive measures are taken depending on the clinical situation. Its symptoms include nausea, vomiting, diarrhea, lack of appetite, lethargy, muscle cramps etc. Sometimes, more serious symptoms are there like heart problems, seizures. Tumor lysis syndrome (TLS) is a medical emergency, if severe, and must be promptly treated.
8. Some other, less common, complications are:
    1. Cardiotoxicity or damage to heart.
    2. Neurotoxicity or damage to nerves.
    3. Infertility.
    4. Increased risk of some types of cancer, especially due to doxorubicin, although the risk is very low.

I have provided an overview of the complications, patients must have detailed discussion about the complications of chemoimmunotherapy with their healthcare providers.

Q. What do you mean by active surveillance?

Answer: if active surveillance is chosen for you, then it means that you don't have to take any treatment (chemo or radiation), you have to undergo periodic evaluation. Active surveillance is different from "observation"; active surveillance uses a battery of tests (the frequency of which is determined by an oncologist experienced in this matter). The goal of active surveillance is to detect progression of disease as early as possible, so that the opportunity of treatment is not missed. The rationale behind active surveillance is that NLPHL is a very slowly growing malignancy and some patients may not require treatment for very long periods of time. Thus, with active surveillance unnecessary toxicity may be avoided and treatment can be initiated only when the disease becomes problematic.

Q. I have completed chemoimmunotherapy (and/or ISRT) for NLPHL. How will the response of therapy be evaluated? How can I be sure that the NLPHL is gone?

Answer: as we have already discussed, chemoimmunotherapy, immunotherapy alone, ISRT or a combination of these may be used for the treatment of NLPHL. After completion of the course of treatment, response evaluation is done.

Following are the components of the response evaluation:
1. Medical history
2. Physical examination
3. Blood tests
4. And most importantly, a PET-CT.

Note that the PET-CT is done:
1. Six to eight weeks after finishing chemotherapy (if only chemotherapy was used for treatment) OR
2. Eight to twelve weeks after finishing radiation therapy.

The goal of NLPHL treatment is "CR" or complete response, also called complete remission. The definition of CR requires that all of the following criteria are met:
1. History and physical examination reveal no evidence of disease or disease-related symptoms.
2. There is no "increased uptake" on PET. This requires some explanation. If we only do a CT scan (without PET), it may still show some lymph nodes which are enlarged (abnormal), after the completion of treatment. But these abnormal appearing lymph nodes may not have residual cancer in them. Doing a PET-CT not only provides us the

anatomic details of lymph nodes, and other organs, but also the "uptake" within them. If the lymph nodes, for example, "light up" on a PET-CT, it means that cancer is still present and if they don't light up, it means that the abnormality is only anatomical, there is no residual cancer.
3. If a bone marrow biopsy was done before starting treatment and it was positive, then it must be negative to be classified as complete response.

Q. I have achieved complete response after my planned course of treatment. What should be done next?

Answer: congratulations, you have achieved CR, now your treatment is complete. Note that:
1. There is no role of any maintenance therapy after CR in NLPHL. You don't need to take any drugs, for NLPHL, once the planned course has been completed and you have achieved CR.
2. For NLPHL, there is no role of stem cell transplant, also colloquially called BMT, in the first CR.

What you do have to go through is surveillance. Surveillance is done for two basic reasons:
1. To monitor treatment complications.

2. To detect possible relapse.

The frequency of visits is not strictly defined, it depends on the clinical situation and the preference of the doctor and the patient. History and physical examination are a must at every visit but the role of imaging tests is not very significant.

Remember:
1. Performing CT scans very frequently is not likely to impact outcomes in case of relapse. Besides, CT scans lead to radiation exposure, which leads to more harm than good in long term. Studies show that relapse is often first detected based on symptoms and physical examination findings rather than CT scans.
2. PET-CT or PET alone has no role in long term surveillance of otherwise healthy patients on follow up.

A point to remember here is that most cases of relapse occur within the first two years of completion of treatment. So, that's the time the patients have to be very vigilant of any symptoms. After two years, the chances of relapse fall, although surveillance is still continued with increasing intervals.

Q. I have completed my planned course of treatment, but the doctors told me that I haven't achieved a complete response. What does it mean and what should I do next?

Answer: the goal is to achieve complete response, but if CR is not achieved, it is not good news. If CR is not achieved then the NLPHL is considered "refractory". Please remember that some patients with refractory NLPHL may be considered for "wait-and-watch" approach, without any active treatment. We will discuss the treatment of refractory NLPHL requiring treatment in the next question.

Q. How is refractory NLPHL treated? (How is relapsed NLPHL treated?)

Answer: the treatment of relapsed or recurrent NLPHL (NLPHL that comes back after initially getting totally cured) and refractory NLPHL (NLPHL that did not attain CR after the first course of treatment, in other words never attained CR), is complex. The treatment decision making is not straightforward, and depends on many factors, like age of the patient, previous therapy and underlying comorbidities. Please discuss about the most appropriate treatment in your case with your oncologist. An important point to remember is that biopsy should be performed again in patient with refractory or relapsed NLPHL because sometimes NLPHL "transforms" into a more aggressive type of lymphoma (for example, DLBCL).

ABOUT THE AUTHOR

Dr. Bhratri Bhushan

Dr. Bhratri Bhushan MBBS, MD (Internal medicine), DM (Medical oncology) is a consultant medical oncologist and hematologist. He has published many books on the subject of oncology and his papers have been published in renowned journals of medical literature. Many of his books have been bestsellers. His works can be found at his AuthorCental page: amazon.com/author/bhratribhushan

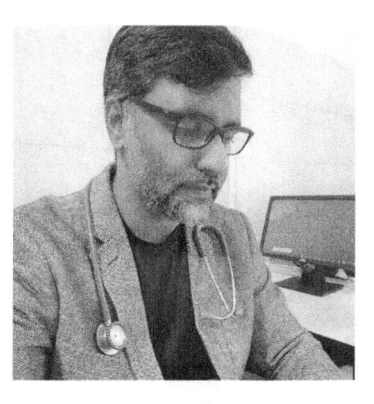

Printed in Great Britain
by Amazon